Lost for Words

Decline int

David

GW01464256

Halo like came
late grief right
conversation Now loss
room now Regret
mother XV time
emotion might assault comfort Dementia story retreat often
difficult just better sadness keep XVII
hand shut life death Home
happy love visit Babble smile
past wait away share make
take door home
fog XVII long Mum lonely Time
guilt find waiting meet interest first
want last one memories tea looking emptiness eagerly
come cruel days Words call
told comes good ask Defying peace something younger became anxious
sisters seem put sound get need watch
feeling Calling Like pain
written answer report much feel
Sitting Greeting Good breathing Patience interested
eyes times situation help
page lost years XII family person Family
communion back bed
older hard grey human names
slow made old everything care
expect everything news control must name
look words see end battle
XXII observe
understand Across steady Resting

Lost for Words
Decline into Dementia

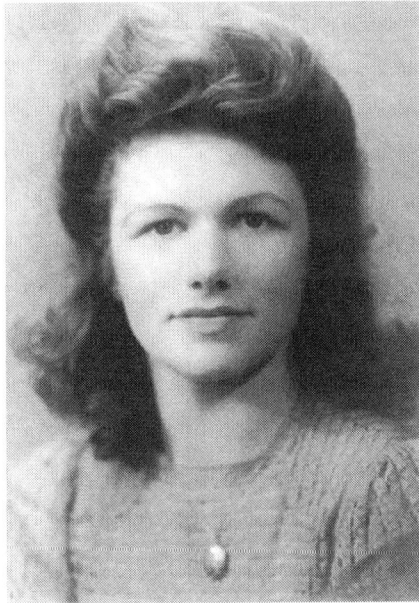

1939

© David Potter, 2014 & 2017

*Dedicated to the memory of my Mother and Father,
Winifred Anglin (1922-2014) and Leonard Potter (1922-2010)
and for all who suffer from dementia and its effects.*

Lost for Words
Decline into Dementia

Introduction

These poems were written after my mother took up full time residence in a care home a few months after my father died in 2010. The poems are a kind of witness to the emotions and episodes experienced over the period until her death in 2014.

Early signs of dementia had been diagnosed in my mother several years previously and we had all witnessed the steady decline in her interest in reading, writing, craft work and conversation. Her memory and her personality all slowly, but surely, slipping away.

It became difficult to communicate with my mother but I have no doubt that she missed my father greatly and that this pain stayed with her all the time, adding to her anxiety.

In the last two years of her life she had several emergency visits to hospital, following falls or infections. This increasing frailty, combined with her depression and dementia, distressed my mother and all who loved her.

These poems record my own guilt and grief for my mother, her suffering, her care and her passing.

It might be that these poems strike a chord with other families facing similar situations where loved ones are descending into dementia, lost for words.

David Potter
July 2014 (revised, January 2017)

I   Visiting Mum in the Care Home

Here to sit and wait
for the words of loss
and emptiness.
For a stuttering conversation,
returning to the same
point of departure.

A bitter calmness and
no resolve or energy
to make it better.
Startled but mute
you stare at me and struggle
for awhile.

On a routine
you do not understand
or want.
You eat your cake
and spill your tea.

Now drifting into sleep
your body at rest
and your breathing steady.
Your eyes beneath their lids
look out on other times
tight shut to keep the happiness within.

Waiting for the correct moment
to say 'goodbye' and
'see you soon'.
I notice you are more agitated,
hovering between dreams and
the harsh reality of here.

II   Greeting Card

I handed her the pen,
she who had once taught me to write.
It's point hovered over the page,
hesitating to make contact with the surface.

Focusing hard, she starts to craft her name.
A seismic line begins to travel in minute detail,
A tremble, meandering across the card.
Once there would have been a flourish,
a neat letter to a friend or sister
eagerly written and eagerly received.
When communication was so much easier.
You seem mildly annoyed,
when I say: 'you have finished'
and take the card away.

III   Words before Dementia

Write sadness on the page
And read it out to me.

Write down this anxiety,
Make it a pretty sentence
To share in your letter.

Resolve this pain
Into words and promises
That they will understand
My sense of loss,
And pain and emptiness.

Do not ask for my opinion
Or expect me to choose.

Just put right this sadness in me.

Help me to find the words,
To put me back to where I was,
to where I was before words stopped,
words before dementia..

IV   Whose Voice?

Whose voice is this?
My mother's voice,
Interpreted from her silence,
Or my own thoughts
Put into words?

There is peace in the
Quietness of our communion.
As you stare at the ceiling
And follow the shadows
On the plaster.
Are you looking for something?

I ask what you see
But, of course, there is
No answer.
So, when I ask if you
Would like some tea,
I am surprised
When you reply,
'Yes please'.

Beside your bed,
It is like sitting
In a waiting room,
Expecting something
To happen.
Is it just for the arrival
Of tea or
Something greater?

When my visit comes
To an end,
I feel we are both
Still waiting.

V   Antique Roadshow

Sitting beside your bed this afternoon
I am wondering if I can
rediscover you.
Like an old master that has been hidden,
over-painted by others,
I am trying to get back to the original.

The canvas of your life
has been cruelly treated of late.
Time spent in the care home,
a growing dependence on others;
your loss, your illness and distressing frailty.
Can I now gently brush away these stains,
with my tears,
or does it need a deeper cleaning?
If I carefully scrub these ugly trials away,
what will I find?
Your younger days, your work days,
your married days and family,
before the long decline.

Your four sisters and your husband
were especially important,
as a network of support
and shared experience.
But time and death has separated you from them
and left you waiting and wanting,
lonely and staring.

As if that past life of vitality and interest
had been discarded and forgotten,
sent off to some jumble sale..
And now I try to peel back the obscuring layers,
to see if there is still the old treasure
of a work of art to be cherished.

VI   Calling Out a Name

Calling out a name
and then something else
I did not catch.

Is he coming to visit?
Will he find his way
to the ward and the bed?

It is not clear to me
who you are summoning up,
who you expect to see.

Who now might hear your call
and hurry down the corridor
to meet your insistence.

Could I hope for some spiritual longing?
a readiness to receive
even in this late hour.

Perhaps you are thinking of Dad,
your faithful tireless companion,
so sadly missed.

A call for someone
to calm you and reassure you
that everything will be alright.

Three kisses for you,
on this difficult
and lonely night.

VII   Eyebrows

It was not until
I saw you lying
on the hospital bed
that I realised,
we have the same eyebrows.
Seeing this,
diverted my eyes
from your oxygen mask,
strapped deeply
over your mouth and nose.
And your grey hair,
thin and crazy
on your pale head.
And the sound of
your ragged breathing.
How you must have battled
with those thick eyebrows
over the years.
To keep them trim
and under control.
Now your breathing
is another battle
and you must struggle
to keep it trim
and under control.

VIII   The Tunnel

I feed you spoonfuls
One by one, as I know
You once did for me.
You doze between each
Helping of soft food,
Dreaming of elsewhere.
Remember those times
When the spoon became a train,
Travelling into the tunnel.
I watch and share
These anxious times,
Open wide.
Through what tunnel
Are you now passing?
How long will be the journey?

IX   Exit

The front door at the care home
Always pulls itself shut,
With a sharp tug and a loud bang.
It comes as a shock
However carefully
You close the door when
You leave the building.
It just takes over
For the last few inches
And slams shut, with a vengeance.

Leaving as quietly as possible,
Trying not to feel guilty
At the end of my visit,
The front door will catch me out again,
And announce my retreat,
With loud disgust.

X   Exchange

The first time I remember seeing
my mother cry, I was six years old.
She was sitting at the foot of the stairs
having just answered the telephone call
that told her, her mother had died.

Standing at the foot of your bed,
these memories come back to me.
I could not then comprehend
the sadness you felt.
I did not know how to console you.

It is a long time ago.
I only have vague memories of my grandmother.
How she spent her last bewildering years,
where you took me to visit her,
how she sometimes came to our house for Sunday lunch.

You must have found it very difficult,
loosing touch with your mother
as she declined into the institution.
And then that feeling of sadness and guilt
when the news came through.

But I cannot ask you about this now.
It is too late to share such memories
And compare the experience of loss and grief.
To exchange notes on the separation
caused by dementia and decline.

XI   A Change

The month has changed.
Outside the birds are singing,
As if Spring has begun.
The snowdrops are early in flower
And the daffodils in bud
But in here, for the first time,
You do not seem to recognise me.

Resting in bed
You might be dozing,
But you have one eye partly open
So I cannot really tell.
You are still and make no sound,
In this changing season.

XII   This Time

This time, you were brighter and more 'with it',
A change from my last recent visit.
It came as quite a shock,
And set me back.
I was unsettled by your temporary engagement.

You seemed more aware of your situation
The paucity of human contact
The hunger and thirst of being left alone too long
Marooned in your bedroom
No bell for you to ring
The door shut on your calling.

The injustice of it all made more stark
By you seeming a little better.
A cruel reward for us both.

XIII   Patience

You are quiet today,
Lying on your back in bed and feeling sleepy.
On the TV, ice hockey from the Olympics
Is pretending to keep you company.
I take the opportunity to look through your daily progress
sheets.
The days punctuated by regular visits from the carers,
Turning you, feeding you, keeping you clean and dry.
The timetabled face of caring.

Sometimes, like buses, the help comes all at once,
But, more often, you have to wait and wait.

You need to learn how to wait,
How to use up time, as you get older.

Patience was never one of Mum's strong points
But now, there is no alternative.
The years tumble but each minute crawls by.

XIV   Like Fog

Dementia is like fog,
drifting over the memory
of people and places.
Rubbing out confidence,
obscuring sight and sound,
and disorientating conversation.
If the wind changes,
the fog's cold embrace
might shift for a while,
and reveal a more familiar shape,
to allow a glimpse of recognition
and remembrance.
But there is no real escape.
As a small patch opens,
the fog builds up elsewhere
and cruelly moves to obliterate
some apparent certainty
that, only yesterday,
brought comfort
to the visitor and companion.

I have lost the person,
who could have put names to the people
in the faded photo,
who could have confirmed those dates
and relationships,
who could have recited the family stories
of older generations,
who could have told me about my childhood days
and put it all in context,
I have lost the person,
to the fog of Dementia.

XV   Untidy Halo

There is a stillness
And relaxed resignation
To the position you adopt,
Lying on your back,
Sleeping.
Your mouth flung half open,
Like a crooked scar
Across your face.
Your white hair
An untidy halo
Around your head,
Resting on the green pillow.

XVI   Defying Gravity

If this poem was you
and it became the
days,
weeks,
months
of your life,
I would not want it to end.
The verse would be uplifting and positive
Moving you over the page in a graceful waltz,
Taking you to all the good and happy memories.
Describing the garden and each flower in detail,
Feeding the horses with fallen apples,
A walk in Valentines Park
And a cup of tea at Lyons Corner House.
Christmas time with brothers and sisters,
A holiday at Margate or Ventnor.
Enjoying the past and looking forward,
Sitting with your grandchildren.
And I would talk about what I could see in your room;
The pictures and photographs,
Letters and cards.
Read extracts from a newspaper,
Recite a poem by Pam Ayres,
Try a Psalm or two.
Babble on about the weather
And the family.
Babble on,
Not stopping the words,
Rising up and defying gravity.

XVII   Regret

I anticipate that,
someday,
perhaps quite soon,
I will regret
not having visited you
more often.
Not entered into more conversations,
albeit one-sided.
Not brought you more news
and gifts and flowers.
I anticipate this future
with a feeling of guilt and remorse,
helpless to respond.
Observing,
to some degree,
I am already
grief stricken.

XVIII   Breaking News

It's breaking news
And I am here to report on the unfolding story.
Full of human interest
It could be a crisis faced by any one of us.
A roller coaster of emotion
To be brutal, it's a life and death situation.
It's got everything
Family drama, personal battle, courage and love.
I observe the enemy's cruel assault,
And watch the slow retreat,
See resistance slipping away.
It's hard not to get upset.

I file my story, my eyewitness report.

It's hard not to get upset,
See resistance slipping away
And watch the slow retreat.
I observe the enemy's cruel assault
Family drama, personal battle, courage and love.
It's got everything,
To be brutal, it's a life and death situation.
A roller coaster of emotion
It could be a crisis faced by any one of us.
Full of human interest
And I am here to report on the unfolding story.
It's breaking news.

XIX   Breathing Out

The bed is a solid metal frame
Adjustable in all planes,
To be raised or tilted,
Lowered or wheeled away.
And the mattress
Well made and comfortable,
Filled with air
To reduce the risk of bed sores.
The room light and airy
The sound of the machine
Pumping fluids down the tube.
The blue cover and the white sheet
Pillows nicely plumped
Oxygen mask securely fixed
Tubes in and out
Pale and poorly.
How much longer,
The steady push of breathing out?

XX   Good

When we get there,
Mum is in bed.
"Am I good?" she asks, "Good?"
Where does that come from, I wonder.
And what answer does she expect?
At first, I think perhaps she means herself,
Well behaved, doing the right thing.
A good person.
Good at the different roles life has put her way.
A good daughter, sister, friend, wife, mother?
But no, it seems to be more a question about her health
And the comfort of where she is.
Her bed, her room, her care.
"Good?"
Does she look well, contented or happy,
In her agitated state?
She clings to my hand.
Can I interpret her meaning more kindly,
Calm her
And give a satisfactory reply?
Does she mean: 'am I ready?'
Ready to get up, ready to go out
Ready to move on.
Good to go back to how everything was before,
Before it all went wrong?
Take my hand, I want to lead you there.
Back to before the falls,
Before the loss of love and confidence,
When you were interested and patient,
Wise and homely.
In control of your world.
Take my hand, mum,
You look lost.

XXI   Photographs

I bring photographs to help the conversation.
Of some recent date,
Great grandchildren having fun,
They smile out in their innocence and beauty.
Mum stares at the images and says
'When can I see them?'
And then there are the other photos
Of an older vintage, with a younger you.
People you named a few months ago
Are now a mystery.
You doubt the names and places I give them
And deny the exotic past I put you in.
You need to have patience for family history
And today you are not interested
In looking backwards.
More
'When can I see them?'

XXII   It should be better than this

No saucers for the cups of tea
No plates for the cakes handed round
No good taste, no quality, no respect.

There is a testiness in the air,
Sparks of mock aggression and silliness,
Across the table, over the cold tea.

It should be better than this,
More humanity and goodness,
No fruit in the bowl, no time to chat.

More annoying, more time wasting,
Difficult and pointless.
The consequence of less engagement.

Everyone is on edge,
A painful balance and pit of anxiety
Present in the residents' lounge this afternoon.

XXIII Until now

Until I had written down these silences between us
I did not realise our communion had no authority,
No authenticity.
Reading back that time, I can now see
The truth and reality of the emotion
Of your despair.
At this distance, I can observe more clearly
The sadness in your eyes and the fear
Of my departing.
Comfortable and cushioned by the time that has passed,
I can worry about the justice of your situation
And sentence.
Safe after my retreat from your bedside,
I can feel the empty hours and lonely days of your waiting,
And grieve.
And this feeling will linger with me until we next meet,
Infect the time and duration when we next sit against the day
And wait.
For the delayed reaction and slow dawning
Of a new understanding, hard won,
And lightly lost.

XXIV Now you are old

Now you are old and grey and full of care
And anxious before me, forgive this verse
And put away the pain and grief you nurse
To find the story that you need to share.

Left lost for words and lonely in this place
Forgetful of those happy days now gone
Hand me your memory to sing your song
And bring to peace your turmoil with glad grace.

When I see your sweet smile break the surface
Not just a backward glimpse of happiness
But something to be thankful for and bless
As, hanging on to love, it will suffice.

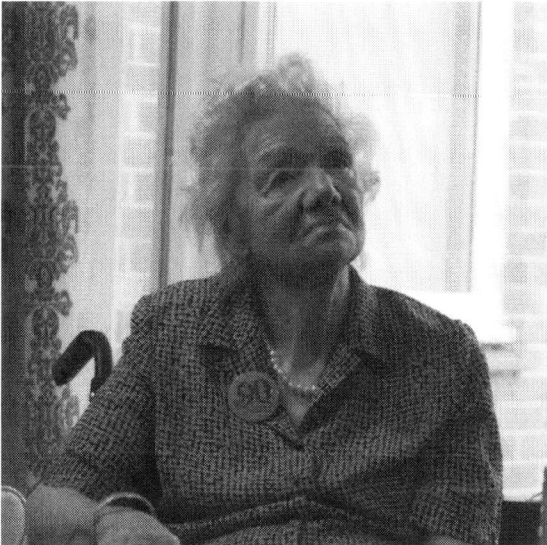

2012

XXV Goodbye

You look frighteningly pale
Your half closed eyes are vacant
You are, perhaps, concentrating
On this final journey.
I joke about a roast-beef drip in your arm
But there is no humour in it
Just my own nervous reaction
To an appalling situation.
I hold your hand
But it is clammy and unresponsive

Your eyes are like misty glass
But seeing nothing.
Breathing is painfully laboured
Rapid and urgent
Scooping up air
Over the white counterpane.
You slightly turn your head
To hear a spoken word
But there is no other recognition
You do not know me now

Later, your eyes are closed
And you are settled into your pillows
Your sagging mouth is open
But your breathing is less violent
Your silver hair has been brushed back
You have been disconnected from
Any feed or drugs
Just staying comfortable.
I bend to kiss your forehead
And say goodbye.

Printed in Great Britain
by Amazon